NUMBER 559

THE ENGLISH EXPERIENCE

ITS RECORD IN EARLY PRINTED BOOKS
PUBLISHED IN FACSIMILE

The publishers acknowledge their gratitude to
the Curators of the Bodleian Library, Oxford
for their permission to reproduce the
Library's copy, Shelfmark: B.2.14.Linc(4)
and to the Trustees of the British Museum
for their permission to reproduce leave C4
from the Library's copy, Shelfmark: 1038.i.38

S.T.C.No. 23612

Collation: A-C^4

Published in 1973 by

Theatrum Orbis Terrarum Ltd.,
O.Z. Voorburgwal 85, Amsterdam

&

Da Capo Press Inc.
- a subsidiary of Plenum Publishing Corporation -
277 West 17th Street, New York N.Y. 1011

Printed in the Netherlands

ISBN 90 221 0559 8

Library of Congress Catalog Card Number:
72-6032

AN ADVICE HOVV TO PLANT TO-BACCO IN ENGLAND:

AND

How to bring it to colour and *perfection, to whom it may be profita-*ble, and to whom harmfull.

*The vertues of the Hearbe in gene-*rall, as well in the outward application as taken in FVME.

WITH

THE DANGER OF THE SPANISH TOBACCO.

Written by C. T.

LONDON,
Printed by NICHOLAS OKES, and are to bee sold by WALTER BVRRE.
1615.

AN ADVICE HOW TO PLANT TOBACCO IN ENGLAND, AND HOW TO BRING IT TO THE COLOVR AND PERfection, to whom it may bee profitable, and to whom *harmefull.*

I Haue heard it reported, by men of good iudgment, that there is paid out of England and Ireland, neere the value of two hundred thouſand pounds euery yeare for Tobacco; and that the greateſt part thereof is bought for ready money. Sure I am, that when our Engliſhmen for theſe ſeuen or eight yeares laſt paſt, traded for it at *Trinidado*, or in *Ore-*

noque, that great ſtore of Gold, Siluer, Coine, and plate was carried hence, and giuen to the Spaniard there in exchange. For ſo greedy were our Engliſh of the Indian Tobacco; as where in the beginning of our traffique there, ſome yeares ſince, the Spaniards (as in all new plantations) were preſt with all ſorts of wants; & had neither cloathes to couer them, nor ſhooes to tread on, nor bread to eate; and did therefore exchange their Tobacco for Fiſh, Wine, Aqua-vitæ, all ſorts of laſting food, for woollen ſtockins, hats, threed, hatchets, & the like: they became in a ſhort time ſo cloyd with all theſe commodities, as nothing (ſome Silkes, and Cloath of Siluer and Gold excepted) but ready Money, and Siluer plate could content them.

This Trade therefore, where the Treaſure of this land is vented for ſmoke, cannot but greatly preiudice the Common-weale: which although it were in ſome ſort tollerable, by reaſon that many ſhippes and Mariners were employed, and that thereby wee kept our knowledge of the Weſt Indies, and bred many ſufficient Marriners: yet ſeeing the Spaniards haue now vtterly baniſhed our Merchants, and put all to the ſword, or to a more cruell death, which they can maiſter, or betray in thoſe parts: I haue thought good, as well for the keeping within the Land of the Treaſure before ſpoken of, then carried into the Indies, and now into

Spaine,

Spaine, as for other respects hereafter remembred; to instruct those of our Nation how to sow, plant and perfect this drugge.

For besides the ill exchange made for this fantasticall merchandize, and besides, the extreame rate, and price of the Indian Tobacco; of which the greatest part is sold for ten times the value of pepper, and the best of it, weight for weight, for the finest siluer; it is hard to find one pound weight in fiue hundred, that is not sophisticate. The blacke colour which it hath, and for which our Shoppe-keepers praise it, is Artificiall: yea all the Tobacco (the leaues of Hispaniola excepted, which wee call Saint *Domingo* Tobacco) is noynted and slubbered ouer with a kinde of iuyce, or syrope, made of Saltwater, of the dregges or filth of Sugar, called *Malasses*, of blacke honey, Guiana pepper, and leeze of Wine; to which in some places they adde a red berry called *Anotto*, and other tawni Berries, with which the Indians paint their bodies, and their beds. This they doe to giue it colour and glosse, to make it the more merchantable, and to giue one and the same countenance to all their rotten, withered, & groundleaues, which they wrappe vp in the midle of their wreathes, couering them ouer on the outside with one that is good.

Of this Tobacco, painted with vnwholsome Berries, there hath beene great store brought into England of late, in which the rednesse and

Art

Art was manifest: so hath there beene vented a kinde of filthy leafe, sold by the Portugalles residing in London, the same beeing made vp in rolles of pounds and halfe pounds.

By these Aditaments is the nature and operation of the Tobacco changed; and the Hearbe made vnhealthfull, and extreame dangerous: for it is well knowne, that how wholsome and medicinable soeuer hunnie it selfe may bee, yet the water of hunnie is starke poyson; and although Indian Pepper, scumme of Sugar, or the dregges or leeze of Wine, and the rest, may be wholesome enough some way vsed: yet to take them into the head in fume, cannot but bee greatly offensiue and preiudiciall. But this is not the worst: for since the Spaniards haue obserued, that the *English* respect but two things chiefly in Tobacco, to wit, the colour, and the biting in the nose, they haue added poyson to the painting, and annoynted the leaues of their Tobacco with common sublimate; by which, though it doe not worke at the instant; yet may the one halfe of all the Gentlemen of England, and many thousands of others be easily poysoned in one yeare.

For it is knowne to many that there hath been Tobacco brought out of Spaine, with dissolued sublimate, which euery man knowes to bee poyson, and no way so dangerously ministred without suspition, as by fume.

The naturall colour of Tobacco is a deepe yellow,

yellow, or a light tawnie: and when the Indians themſelues ſold it vs for Kniues, Hatchets, Beads, Belles, and like merchandiſe, it had no other complexion, as all the Tobacco at this day hath, which is brought from the coaſt of Guiana, from Saint *Vincents*, from Saint *Lucia*, from *Dominica*, and other places, where we buy it but of the naturall people; and all theſe ſorts are cleane, and ſo is that of S^t. *Domingo*, where the Spaniards haue not yet learned the Art of Sophiſtication.

There is alſo a ſort of Caraccas Tobacco, which the Indians make vp, and ſell to the Spaniards, which is wholeſome enough; but there comes little of it into England

Now beſides theſe harmefull mixtures, if our Engliſh which delight in Indian Tobacco, had ſeene how the Spaniſh ſlaues make it vp, how they dreſſe their ſores, and pockie vlcers, with the ſame vnwaſht hands with which they ſlubber and annoynt the Tobacco, and call it ſauce *Per los perros Luteranos*, for *Lutheran* dogges; they would not ſo often draw it into their heads and through their noſes as they doe: yea many a filthy ſauour ſhould they find therein, did not the ſmell of the hunny maiſter it; which ſmell euery man may plainly perceiue that takes of the blacke role Tabacco, brought from *Orenoque*, *Trinidado*, and elſe-where.

To the end therefore, as I haue already ſaid,

that the treaſures exchanged for Tobacco, may be kept within the Land; that thoſe that delight therin may haue it at a better rate, and to auoyd the danger of the Spaniſh mixtures, I haue hereunder ſet downe certaine obſeruations, by the helpe of which all that are diſpoſed to plant Tobacco in England, may aſſuredly bring the ſame to ſtrength and perfection: yea to ſtrength exceeding all that is brought from the Indies.

Now the firſt thing that you are to take care for, muſt be the ſoyle: of which the ground naturally fertile, is the beſt, and that which hath not borne any other but graſſe: for if you ſow your ſeede in ground enriched with dung, except you ſtay two yeare at leaſt, til the dung and the vapour therof be conſumed, your Tobacco will retaine the ſauour of it.

If you ſow it where Cabbage and Turnips haue beene lately ſowne; thoſe rootes will alſo infect your Tobacco with their ſmell. Nay you muſt take care that your ground be not ouer-fat: for the fatteſt grounds bring forth ſo thicke and ſo rugged a leafe, and ſo fild with moyſture, as it will neuer be brought to any colour, neuer to any ſtrength, nor neuer burne well in the pipe: A good ſoyle, neither too rich nor too poore, is the beſt, and the beſt helpe to better the barren, is dung of ſheepe.

The ſeedes which you are to ſowe, are of two kindes, the male and female; the male is the leſ-

ſer

ſer leafe, and beares a yellow flower; of which kinde is that of Braſill, which the people of the land call *Petun*.

The female brings a very large leafe, and farre larger and longer in England, and in France, then in the Indies; by reaſon of their ſandy grounds, and want of raine there; and it beares a pale incarnate flower. If this latter kinde would ripen in England, in certainty it would yeeld farre more profite to the planters, it requireth leſſe labour in the gathering, withering, and making vp: and being ripe, it will come to a perfect tawny colour, without any other Art then the ſtouing: but the leſſer leafe is generally the ſtronger, and ſubiect to leſſe hazard then the greater.

In all the months betweene September and Aprill you may caſt your ſeed into the ground: for as that ſeed which falleth of it ſelfe in the end of September, and lyeth as it falleth vncouered, doth grow and thriue as well as that which is ſowne in Ianuary, February, or March: ſo doth the laſt ſowing in Aprill proſper as well, and grow as ſoone ripe as any of the reſt. When it is ſowne it muſt bee couered but thinly with earth: for if you rake too much earth ouer it, it will come vp too late to ripen for that yeare.

If the Spring bee dry, you muſt water it often to bring it out of the ground: your water muſt be riuer or pond water; for that of welles is too

 cold,

cold, except you ſet it all the day in the Sunne.

After your ſeedes are growne vp to a ſtalke of three inches high, you muſt take them vp and replant them, leauing two foot betweene each plant of the leſſer kinde, and three foote betweene each plant of the greater. If you leaue your plants ſo long on the ground ere you ſet them abroad, that the ſtalke haue ſixe inches in length, then muſt you either bury in the ground foure of the ſixe inches, or elſe they will hang the head, and be long ere they recouer: and hauing ſet them in ſo deepe you bury that part of the ſtalke which would bring out your faireſt and ſtrongeſt leaues: you muſt therefore replant as ſoone as you haue a ſtalke able to be ſet abrode.

You muſt alſo take care to water your plants once a day: in the morning, if the Spring bee cold; in the euening if it bee warme; otherwiſe they will wither, or ſtand long ere they recouer.

After they are growne a foote high, or ſomewhat more, they will offer to knob, and caſt out little buttons for ſeede; which they will doe the ſooner if you ſowe them in the increaſe of the Moone, which you muſt auoyd. Theſe knobbes you muſt euery day nippe off, ſo muſt you doe all the by-branches that it caſteth out, and all the ſtalkes but one that ſhoots out of the ſame root: you muſt leaue but one ſtalke, and vpon it not

aboue

aboue 8 or 10 leaues. This pruning must be continued from the time that your Tobacco begins to yeeld shuttes and buttons for seed, euen to the time that you gather it: which if you shall neglect, coueting to haue many stalkes, because many leaues, your Tobacco will be weake and worth nothing.

Your next and greatest care must bee, your patience to attend the ripening: for if you gather your leaues before they change colour on the stalke, they will be good for nothing. Your corne and all other fruits and graines may teach you this, that nothing hath any great vertue where nature is preuented. When your leaues be toward ripening, they will bee full of yellow spottes, which you shal best discerne if you hold a leafe betweene you and the light.

And yet you must not so loue your owne as to take it greene: for if when you cut it and dry it, how strong soeuer it proue in the taking of it, the greatnesse shewes that either it wants ripenesse or fermentation; it must looke yellow at the least, otherwise it may proue equally harmefull with that which is sophisticate. I must also aduise you, not to slubber your English with *Mel rosarum*, and other trumpery, as many of our owne Artificers do, therby to bring it to the Indian colour: it is an impious practise to play with the health of men, and to make profite by their destruction. Your English Tobacco if you giue it time to ripen, and time to ferment, will change colour, and cast off all her naughty and vnwholsome moysture, and change her greene garment for that which is perfect yellow or tawny, without any art or addition.

When you haue gathered the ripe leaues, for all will not be ripe at once, you may lay them in the Sunne for two or three houres, otherwise they will be so brickle, as they will breake in the stringing: and if the weather bee cloudy, then you may leaue them in your baskets two or three dayes, and then string them vpon threed, and so hang them in a close roome, where no winde entreth, or lay them on a cleane boorded floore, till they wither and become yellowish, which they will do in 10, 12, or 14 dayes, but you may not ouer-dry them; for then they will not sweat and change colour.

When they are thus withered, but not dried to crumble, you must stoue them in heapes, in a heat somewhat stronger then a hot-house, and like vnto the heate of an Ouen after the bread drawne: for if your heate bee too great, it will burne, if too little, it will require a long time in their sweating, or fermentation, ere they bee brought to perfection. But if you suffer your leaues to be perfect ripe ere you gather them, then they will ferment in a short time, and obtaine a perfect Indian colour, I meane the naturall Indian colour, though not the artificiall and

blacke.

blacke. He that weares cloath to the end it was inuented for, to wit, to defend him from cold, and wet, cares more for the goodnesse then the colour: howsoeuer it is better to accept of our owne with some little fault, then to vse the India with a great deale of filthinesse.

In the meane time, and vntill we haue store of our owne, I aduise my Countrey-men to take the leafe of Saint *Domingo*, or the leaues of *Dominica*, and of the Ilands adioyning, or those Indian leaues that are of a deep yellow, or slight tawny, which colours are naturall, and forbeare the blacke which is foule, the dyed Tobacco, which is red, and the leafe brought in by the Portugalles, and the like slubbered stuffe.

The Tobacco which comes from the Barmuda is cast away either by neglecting to prune it, or else because they nourish ouer-many leaues on one stalke, which they do either out of Ignorance, or for that they couet to haue the greater quantity, or otherwise; because, as I heare, they imitate the Spaniards in iuicing it: that place would otherwise giue vs that which is excellent, and so would Virginia.

For the rest, after you haue taken your Tobacco out of your stoue, you must lay it abrode some three or foure dayes: for if you make it vp too moist, it will grow mouldy.

For conclusion, because there hath beene much dispute about this hearbe, whether it bee

wholsome

wholſome or harmfull: I will let my Countrey-men know, what by long experience, and conference with others, I finde.

It is taken in all America, euen from Canada to the ſtraights of Magellan, in all Affrica vpon the coaſt, from Barbary to the Cape of good hope, and ſo till you come to the mouth of the red ſea; it is alſo vſed in moſt of all the kingdomes of the Eaſt Indies.

The Spaniards and Indians of the Weſt giue vs three principall reaſons why they vſe it: the firſt is becauſe it opens the body, and lets out the heate by the pores which is *præter naturam* within them: the ſecond is, the conſumption and auoyding of ſuperfluous moyſture wherewith they are filled by eating of fruits abundantly, by drinking of water, and in all the In-land Countries for want of ſalt: the third is, becauſe it ſtaies both hunger and thirſt, and doth refreſh them after great trauaile and toyle: theſe be the general vertues and knowne to all: but the Spaniſh Phyſitians, their Prieſts, and others that are learned, finde ſomewhat elſe, and of more importance in this hearbe: for they vſe a confection of Tobacco in all Callentures or burning feuers, and they take it in ſmoke to defend them in long nauigations from the ſcuruy, and they cure with it all ſores and vlcers: yea it is certaine, that the iuice of Tobacco, mixt with a little ſea-water, doth reſiſt the venome of poyſo-

ned

ned arrowes, wherewith the Spaniards (how ſlight ſoeuer the hurt bee) are without ſuch a help wounded to death. The Braſilians ſay that it is cordiall, and they alſo take it to ſtay hunger and thirſt when they trauel and want ſuſtenance. The people of the South parts of Virginia eſteeme it exceedingly, and ſo doe the reſt: they ſay that God in the creation did firſt make a woman, then a man, thirdly great maize, or Indian wheat, and fourthly, Tobacco: they vſe it for the curing of wounds, and in ſmoke as we doe; and they are ſuperſtitiouſly led to beleeue that when they are in danger of drowning, in foule wether, that if they caſt Tobacco into the water, that the billow will fall, and grow leſſe. *Monardus* the Spaniard commends it in all pains of the head, growing by deſtuctions or windy vapors, in the tooth-ake occaſioned by cold rume, in all diſeaſes of the breaſt, old coughes, aſmaticall paſſions, and the like, in all paines of the ioynts, and ſwellings, if the leaues roaſted vnder imbers be often applied; which the Indian women adminiſter to their children for the coldneſſe of their ſtomacke, and windineſſe. The ſame Author affirmeth, that in the ſuffocation of the matrix, it is a preſent remedie, if the leaues made warme be applied to the nauell or bottome of the belly; in all greene woundes and vlcers, and in the gangrene he prizeth it aboue all other vegetables: yea hee affirmeth that an experience was made in the preſence of *King Philip* the ſecond

L.1.Simplicium medicament.ex nouo orbe dilatorum.

cond of Spaine, vpon a dogge poysoned. These be *Monardus* his words, as I finde them in *Clusius*, *Rex ipse Catholicus, eius vires experiri volens, Cani vulnus infligi iussit in gutture, & toxico quo venerat ores vtuntur, illini; & paulo post foliorum Tobacci succum satis copiose instillari, & ipsa folia trita super vulnus ligari: liberatus est canis non sine omnium admiratione.* The Catholicke King willing to make triall of the vertue of it, caused a dogge to haue a wound made in his throat, and to be anointed with poyson which the hunters vse; and a while after he made the iuyce of Tobacco to bee plentifully powred into it, and the brused leaues to be bound vpon the wound, and the dogge was healed, to the no smal admiration of all that were present. The same Author commends this hearbe for the cure of the *Polypus*, and doth avow that he himselfe hath cured it with the iuice of Tobacco.

Fol. 310. *Clusius* in his experience affirmeth, that in all old vlcers putride, and of a maligne quality, in the gangren, in the scabbes, clouds in the eyes, &c. he hath vsed the vnguent of Tobacco with happy successe.

Mr *Gerald* in his history of plants, or great herball, tels vs, that the dropsie hath been cured with the iuce of Tobacco; and in the same *Fol.* 288. book, he teacheth the cõposition of an vnguent made with the lesser or male Tobacco: which booke, becanse the poorer sort are not able to buy, & that the said *Gerald* doth so highly commend

mend the vse of this hearbe, I thought good to take it out word for word, for the common good of all poore people needing such a remedy, and these be his words. I do make hereof an excellent balsame to cure deepe wounds and punctures, &c. which balsame doth bring vp the flesh from the bottome very speedily, & also heale simple cuts in the flesh, according to the first intention, that is, to glew or soder the lips of the wound together, not procuring matter or corruption vnto it, as is commonly seene in the healing of wounds. Take (saith he) oyle of roses, oyle of Saint *Iohns* wort, of either one pint, the leaues of Tobacco, stamped smal in a stone morter, two pound, boyle them together to the consumption of the iuice, straine it, and put it to the fire againe, adding thereunto of Venice Turpentine two ounces, of Olibanum and Mastic, of either halfe an ounce in most fine and subtill powder, which may at all times make it into an vnguent or salue, by putting therunto wax and rosin, to giue vnto it a stiffe body. He further saith, that the iuice or distilled water of the lesser leafe is very good against catharres, the dizinesse of the head, and rhumes that fall down to the eyes, against the paine called the Migrame, if either you apply it to the temples, or take one or two greene leaues, or the drye leafe moystened in wine, and warmed on Imbers, and apply it. Many notable medicines are made hereof against the old and inueterate cough, a-

 gainst

against asthmaticall and pectorall griefes, which if I should set downe at large, would require a peculiar volume. So farre *Gerald*.

For the taking of it in smoke, if the Tobacco be cleane, and not poysoned with iuices, and other Art, I know that it is an excellent remedy for the head-ake, for the *vertigo* & dizines of the head, for moist & watery stomakes, it preuaileth against the rumes & defluctions, & all the pains of the ioynts therby occasioned, and against all affections of the head, watering of the eyes, and tooth-ake, that it keepes off the gout and sciatica, and taketh away the rednesse of the face, that at sea it preserueth those that take it both from the Calenture or burning Feuer, and from the Scuruie, that it openeth obstructions, and is exceeding profitable in the falling sickenesse. The syrope is a good vomite, and so is a draught of white or renish wine, wherein so much of the leafe as weigheth sixe pence hath beene steeped all night: the oyle that droppeth out of a foule pipe, killeth Tetters, and all of that kinde.

The Hearbalists and other Physitians make diuers kindes or *species* of this Tobacco; they commend that which beareth the great leafe, and pale incarnate flower, and call it the true Tobacco, a second sort they call *Petum*, and a third *Nicosian*.

Others (and thinke they speake learnedly) call our English of the lesser leafe, yellow Henbane, or *Hoscyamus Luteus*; and the greater *Hoscya-*

mus Peruuianus; yea they make a difference between the Tobacco of *Paria* and *Trinidado*, and that of *Peru*; although I am well assured, that there was neuer any one pound of *Peru* Tobacco seene in England or in Europe. But if the hearb which we call Sage, differ in kind from the same hearbe, because the French cal it *Searge*, and the Latines *Saluia*, and so all other hearbs, which diuers nations call diuersly: then doth the *Petum*, the *Nicosian*, and the *Tobacco* differ; otherwise there is nothing between them. But the greatnesse & littlenesse which we distinguish by male and female, as in many other hearbs we doe the like: for the Spaniards which first found this plant in the Isle *Tobaque*, did therfore call it after the name of that Island: and it is true, that because there is no better soile in the world, and that it hath raine & heat sufficient, the Tobacco there growing is very large. Of this very kinde (found euery where in *America*) it was that *Iohn Nicot*, born in *Nismes* in *Languedoc*, & Embassador in Portugall for *Henry* the 2d of France, sent of the seed to Queen *Katherine* of *Medicis*, after called, *Queene Mother of France*, wherevpon it was by some called, *Queene Mothers hearbe*, by others it was and is still called *Nycosian*, and yet *Theuet* vaunts that he sent it into France 10 years before *Nicots* Embassage. Now as the *Brasilians* call this *Tobacco*, *Petum*, so in the *West Indies* it is cald *Vicielt*, saith *Monardus*: and *Ouiedus. lib.* 11 c. 5. saith, that in *Hispaniola* it is cald *Perebecenut*, the

Clusius & Seres
Theuet. Cos. gen.
Simp. Medicam.

the Guianians call it *Tamoi*, other Nations *Tekel*, & the Virginians *Opoak*, & it is euery where, and in England it selfe, greater, according to the soyle: yea it differs in taste, thickenesse, largenesse, and goodnesse almost in euery Garden wherein it is planted.

True it is, notwithstanding that there are found manifest differences in the male and female, or in the greater or the lesse, both in flower & largenesse, though both of one kinde, the same being found in many Hearbes, Plants, and Trees besides.

Now for those that make Tobacco a kinde of *Hoscryamus*, because it stupifieth as *Hoscryamus*, or Henbane doth, they may as wel say that *Opiũ* is also a kinde of Tobacco, or Tobacco a kinde of *Opium*, or that *Stramonium* is of that *species* which benummeth more then either Tobacco or *Opium*. For the rest, this is true, that as it is vsually taken in England, it hath more of the ill then of the good. For those that take Tobacco with wine, do absolutely alter the propertie of it, & make it the Artificer of many ill accidents and diseases, I meane all those that drinke wine betweene meales, and presently after the taking of it. For where God hath giuen this hearbe for a remedy to those poore people that want both wine, spice, and salt, that doe often swim riuers, and diue vnder water, that goe naked, and are beaten with showres, that feed aboundantly vppon fruits, that suffer hunger and thirst, that liue

in

in a region violently hot: we in this part of the world vse Wine of all sorts, and all sorts of Spices, we eate salt with our meat, and powder our flesh and fish with it, and thereby drye vp, and sucke out the corrupt and harmefull moysture that it hath: we that, besides Wine, haue strong Beere, & strong Ale, that couer our bodies with garments, and are prest with cold for three parts of the yeare, do not need any such drying fume at all.

It is true that those that haue decaying bodies, those that are of yeares, and opprest with moysture and fleame, those that are subiect to rhumes and the cough, that haue cold stomackes, and are inclined to the gout, or haue it, or that are subiect to any of the imperfections before named, for those it is a singular remedy. But it destroies all our youth that take it without cause, and euery houre of the day, it makes them tender and not able to endure the aire, it makes them dull and sleepy, brings them to the rhume and tooth-ake, marres their teeth, except they cleanse them often, begets in them a drouth, and consequently a desire to drinke: yea and an entrance to drunkennesse it selfe: for many of them finding some little sickenesse in their stomackes when they take strong Tobacco, do presently drinke of the strongest Wines: the Tobacco opens the body, and makes way, by which the wine inuadeth the liuer, and drieth it vp: yea taken in that manner with strong drinkes it con-

sumes

ſumes the radicall moyſture, and haſtneth on old age: the Indians doe therefore forbid it the children, till they haue taken wiues and haue had children, as wee in England were wont to forbid maides and yong men the vſe of Wine: for though Tobacco ſtirre the appetite, yet is it no friend to generation, vſed with wine as before remembred. He that deſireth further knowledge of this Hearbe, let him reade *Oliuer de Serres, L.* of *Pradel* in his *Agriculture,* and *Car. Stephanus* vpon the ſame ſubiect, *lib.2.c.76.*

FINIS.